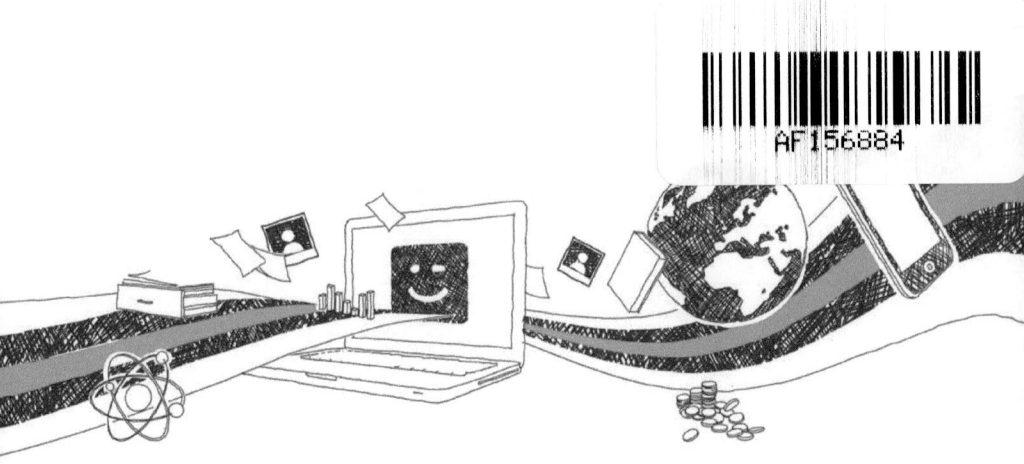
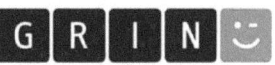

Bibliographic information published by the German National Library:

The German National Library lists this publication in the National Bibliography; detailed bibliographic data are available on the Internet at http://dnb.dnb.de .

Imprint:

Copyright © 2018 GRIN Verlag
Print and binding: Books on Demand GmbH, Norderstedt Germany
ISBN: 9783668931893

This book at GRIN:

https://www.grin.com/document/458156

Ulrich Schmitz

Aus der Reihe: e-fellows.net stipendiaten-wissen

e-fellows.net (Hrsg.)

Band 3091

Challenges of measuring dental service quality

GRIN Verlag

GRIN - Your knowledge has value

Since its foundation in 1998, GRIN has specialized in publishing academic texts by students, college teachers and other academics as e-book and printed book. The website www.grin.com is an ideal platform for presenting term papers, final papers, scientific essays, dissertations and specialist books.

Visit us on the internet:

http://www.grin.com/

http://www.facebook.com/grincom

http://www.twitter.com/grin_com

SERVICE QUALITY AND COMMISSIONING

Challenges of Measuring Dental Service Quality

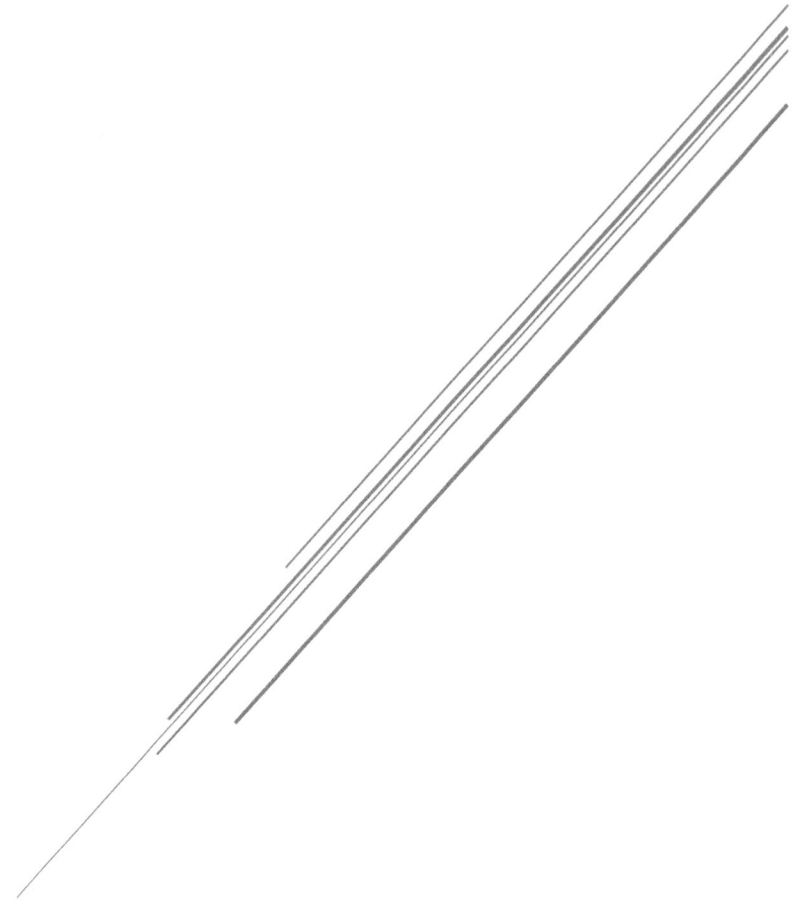

Ulrich Schmitz
Manchester Metropolitan University

Content

Introduction

The aim of this report is to show typical difficulties to measure service quality in healthcare services and to discuss potential approaches offered by science to meet these challenges. The area of "General Dentistry" is chosen as an example for the complexity of services.

Dentistry includes several fields with different specifications.
Main divisions are:
- Prophylaxis and Preventive Dentistry
- Dental examinations
- Orthodontics
- Restorative Dentistry
- Endodontics
- Periodontics
- Prosthetics
- Oral Surgery
- Implantology

A general practitioner may offer all or just selected specifications. As might be expected every division demands completely different strategies to evaluate service and its quality. As distinguished from human medicine dentistry is not separated into countless specialisations, after finishing studies in general dentistry only 3 academic specialisations are offered by universities:
- Orthodontics
- Oral Surgery
- Periodontics

Scientific dental societies provide continuing education on all other fields for general dentists, who perform most of all treatments. This must be kept in mind, because the number of different treatments complicates evaluation of quality.

The first part of this report gives an overview about service, quality, service quality and their definitions.
Then the second part looks at different challenges of measuring the quality from two sides:
- from the perspective of the service provider, the dentist and the team
- from the perspective of the service recipient, the patient and -in any sense- the healthcare insurance company.

To get a better understanding of this distinction differences between quality and performance are explained.
Different requirements and patient expectations on treatments in various subdivisions are outlined.
The third part contains a discussion of methods to measure quality, paying special attention to SERVQUAL:

- Performance targets
- Surveys
- SERVQUAL

As a conclusion the outcomes of those methods may be used as a foundation to get some practical advice to assist a dental office to determine its position in the local market and to identify areas of potential improvements.

Part 1: Overview and Definitions

Service

Before starting to think about measuring "service quality" this should be defined.
What does "service" mean? What is hidden behind "quality"?

Current literature offers several definitions for "service". It is obvious there is no generally accepted one.
A wide definition is given by the BusinessDictionary (businessdictionary.com): "A valuable action, deed, or effort performed to satisfy a need or fulfill a demand."
Translated into dentistry it may look like this: The dental treatment performed by a dental team to satisfy the patient's need for pain-free and healthy teeth or fulfil the demand for aesthetic and cosmetic improvements of a smile.
Primarily that is an explanation of the goal of a service, but no characteristics which distinguish services from goods are included. In 2007 Gronroos introduced a comprehensive definition. Additional key points are:
- Service is a process (may be interpreted as perishability)
- It consists of "more or less intangible activities" (intangibility)
- There may be interactions between customer and employees (inseparability, heterogeneity)
- Service provides solutions to customer problems

The choice of words gives a hint to apply the mentioned additions to a continuum.
They are the most commonly accepted characteristics of a service (Bateson, 1995), known as the IHIP model.

IHIP Model

IHIP is an abbreviation for:

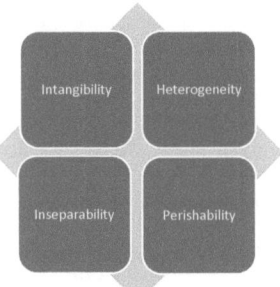

These service characteristics are applied to the dental treatment to explain the weight and need to consider continuums.
- Intangibility
  It is obvious that the dental treatment itself is intangible, but the patient's perception is influenced by tangible elements like the look of equipment and the environment of the practice.

Moreover, dentistry often produces tangible outcomes like fillings and dentures. Taking all these points into account dental treatment may be rated at just 75 % on an intangibility continuum.

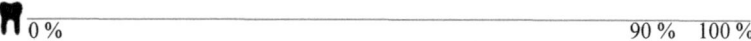

0 %   75 %   100 %

- Heterogeneity
  As patients are humans and no industrial workpieces everyone is different. They have different time frames, different pain thresholds, sometimes additional medical problems, and different expectations. They may be (positive or negative) influenced by family and friends or by internet research.
  For everyone an individual care approach must be found, especially because dentistry appears as a high-contact service (Gronroos, 2007).
  Furthermore, the dentist, assistants, and receptionists are humans, too. The knowledge and mood of every single member, who is involved, may have an important impact on the treatment and its outcome.
  To minimise these effects on the side of the providers there are movements to standardise typical treatments. A routine workflow may be captured as a step-by-step chart.
  But this can only be seen as a kind of technical help with limitations in consideration of different types of patients.
  Therefore, 90 % on a heterogeneity continuum seem to be appropriate.

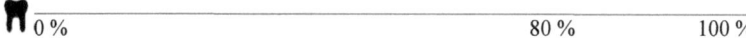

0 %   90 %   100 %

- Inseparability
  For a dental examination or treatment the patient and the dentist have to be at the same place, normally in a treatment room. To work on teeth it must be possible to see and touch them.
  But again, there may appear some exceptions in dentistry:
    o A lot of work is done in laboratories. Here plaster models of the patient's teeth are basis for the making of crowns, bridgeworks, and prostheses.
    o After taking x-rays the patient's presence is not necessary to analyse them.
    o Prescriptions may be written and sent to the patient by mail.
  Even inseparability doesn't reach 100 % on its continuum, 80 % is a reasonable choice.

0 %   80 %   100 %

- Perishability
  Parallels with intangibility may be detected.
  Each treatment is consumed directly, storage isn't possible, but the outcomes should last for a longer time. Fillings and lab work have to stay in mouth for several years. In Germany a practice has to give a 2-year-guarantee on every work, replacements within this time aren't paid by insurance companies.
  That's why 75 % on the perishability continuum are a good fit.

0 %   75 %   100 %

After this integration of dentistry into the context of "service" the second term "quality" is evaluated.

Quality

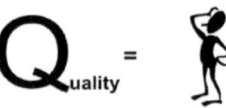

$$Q_{uality} =$$ (youtube.com, Sood, M., 2013)

"Even though quality cannot be defined, you know what it is." (Pirsig, R., 1976)

That transcendent approach makes it difficult to know how to satisfy as it refers to an innate quality of excellence (Shirley, D., 2011). Unfortunately, in dentistry most patients act in that way. As there is no universal idea of quality, everyone has an own one. This leads to challenges, which are discussed later.

There are several other approaches (Garvin, 1983), which are applied by different stakeholders.

User-based (patient view)	Quality "lies in the eyes of the beholder", but many users share their view based on "market" demand (Shirley, D., 2011). Modern technology enables fast and wide sharing of this perceived quality in social networks and especially on rating platforms. A dentist or a clinic with many good ratings is perceived as a provider of good quality by potential patients.
Value-based (patient or dentist view)	Price is the critical factor in this case. If no other information is available this may be a pivotal quality indicator (Zeithaml, 1981). The costs for dental treatment are set by the government fixing the scale of fees (German "BEMA"). Primary care is covered by the statutory health insurance, but patients may pay an additional fee for "better" filling materials like composites and must pay about 40 % of every treatment in prosthodontics. There are extreme price differences between dentists. The patient has to decide which offer fits best for her/him. On the other hand, the dentist has to think about the price to charge. It may be a decision about what quality will be offered or which kind of patients ought to be addressed.
Manufacturing-based (dentist view, marketing)	"Quality means conformance to requirements" (Crosby, 1979; Shirley, D., 2011). The crucial point is measurement. That is helpful in manufacturing products, where specifications are measurable. In dentistry, just procedures are measurable against a process protocol, which can be created by the dentist or a specialist, plus auxiliary specialities like hygiene where outcomes of sterilisation have to be logged. Some practices acquired an ISO certification to showcase

	constant quality. However, the requirements to measure against are not published. Thus, the process protocol itself may not represent "state of the art", though its heeding will be certified.
Product-based (insurance company view)	This approach measures quality from the side of the output. It is an easy way as outcomes can be compared with set specifications (Gronroos, 1990). It should be noted that it, too, works well with the production of goods, but "knowledge about goods quality is insufficient to understand service quality" (Parasuraman et al., 1985).

Table 1a - d

German insurance companies use this approach as a questionable way to reduce their costs. With assistance of the government rules for guarantees on dental work were legislated. It was set that renewable fillings and prostheses aren't chargeable again within two years. In this way dental treatment is reduced to a measurable product, which has to last at least for two years, without taking any special features or patients' medical problems into account.

Though this report concentrates on the stakeholder patient and dentist, the different approaches to quality demonstrate, that there are more interested parties with different ideas involved to be considered.

Service Quality

The different approaches to quality require various definitions of service quality, too. As expressed above every stakeholder uses an own view belonging to their personal interests. In addition, especially patients are no homogeneous group. Therefore, it is nearly not possible to find a universal definition. A broad one by Kotler and Armstrong (1996) sees service quality as "the totality of features and characteristics of a product or service that bear on its ability to satisfy stated or implied needs". It is usable for the service "dentistry", but the value of offered features and characteristics is in the eye of the beholder.
With other words: Service quality is everything a patient individually expects.

Though it is possible to work dentistry out as a service, there is no way to give a definition of dental quality, which is universally applicable.
Thus, before evaluation of service quality the investigator and her/his intentions as well as the recipients must be known. It is important for all participants to have a clear and equal understanding of service quality.
Misunderstandings and problems will occur, if different stakeholders with different ideas of quality have to negotiate without an agreement on their definitions in advance.

One already mentioned example for such a misunderstanding are negotiations about the dental remuneration of statutory insurance companies. With a little more interest in all stakeholders' views and a focus on the patient's needs the product-based approach to quality wouldn't be legally defined.
Similar problems even occur on a lower level when the number of stakeholders is reduced from 5 (politics, insurance companies, industry, dentists, patients) to 2 (dentist – patient).

Every patient (and dentist) has her/his own vision of service quality.
The heterogeneity of patients induces various individual assumptions to reach satisfaction, but service quality should be consistent through most of the interactions.
Dentists may follow a guideline given by their professional organisations. The STEEEP model by the Dental Quality Alliance (DQA), part of the American Dental Association (ADA) is a good example (DQA, 2016):

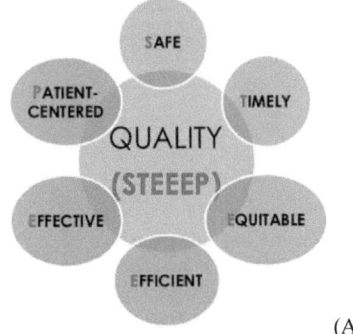

(ADA.org)

Safe	Avoiding injuries
Timely	Reducing waits and delays
Effective	Avoiding underuse and overuse
Efficient	Avoiding waste
Equitable	No vary in quality based on personal characteristics
Patient-centered	Respectful of and responsive to individual needs

Table 2

Patients don't have a professional guideline. They follow individual expectations, influenced by several factors mentioned later.
It's a challenge to match the guided perspective of a dentist with the unguided expectation of a patient.

Part 2: Challenges of Measuring Service Quality

View from the Perspective of the Service Provider

A big challenge for the dentist is **to decide why and what to measure**.
Several reasons could be possible for the need of a deeper look at service quality:
-   Benchmarking of the practice
-   Looking for fields to grow or improve
-   Searching for a reason of patient loss
-   Information to support decisions about investments in new equipment

These are examples from different fields to demonstrate the necessity of a well-chosen subject to measure.

Benchmarking

If benchmarking is the main goal, only published data could be compared with own collected data. A look at the statistical yearbook 2017 of the professional body "KZBV (Kassenzahnärztliche Bundesvereinigung)" leads the way to the best choice.

Typically, a well- educated and -trained dentist wants to achieve best state-of-the -art outcomes due to several reasons:

- Professional behaviour
- Meeting patients' expectations
- Marketing and competition
- Target of insurance companies

Thus, one option is the measurement of outcomes.

Several objective data are conceivable:

- Marginal leakage of crowns and bridgework
- Stability of fillings and prostheses
- Repetition rate of fillings
- Number of repeated visits
- Number of patients treated per day or month

Own results may easily be compared with published overall data and a personal classification is possible.

Taking only such external factors into consideration may be helpful to create a foundation of minimal requirements to be met, but leaves out the wide field of subjective factors, both in patients and providers.

As these factors aren't comparable or released, benchmarking has to be confined to performance data.

This is the right place to introduce the conceptual pair:

Performance – Service Quality

"How well a person, machine, etc, does a piece of work or an activity", the Cambridge Dictionary defines "performance". It is an easy to measure, objective factor, which may vary from day to day, patient to patient. It is the outcome, that is paid by insurance companies. As this is the only objective part there are trends to use it as the only value to determine service quality in health care.

Such a concept may work well in an industrial environment to rate production.

- Building 10 products A each day is a better performance than 9 products A. The first worker or machine is the better choice.
- Performing 10 Composite-fillings each day is a better performance than 9 fillings?

This question cannot be answered easily, because a lot of information - primarily about the patient - is missing. "Soft" elements on both sides, like attitude, building relationships, and behaviour of the dentist and assistants as well as fear, expectations, and possible medical problems of the patient are hidden.

Reducing service quality to performance leaves at least interaction, physical environment, and patients' expectations aside.

Improvement

If the practice looks for fields to improve, performance data may be helpful, but there are several other "soft" factors to grow, which may establish a competitive advantage over many dental offices.

As performance data can easily be collected and analysed, it is a challenge to choose and measure a suitable "soft" factor.

Some of them are:

- To take enough time for every patient
- To listen to the patient's needs
- To work as painless as possible
- To build personal relationships with long-term patients

After a decision for one or more factors to improve in, an appropriate way to measure has to be chosen. As there are no objective numbers to count a patient's perception must be taken into account, too. Guidance comes from Baldwin and Sohal (2003), who identified fear and anxiety, appreciation of punctuality, and involvement in the development of treatment plans as significant impacts upon service quality perception.

Patient loss

Today the dental market changes from a demand-driven one to a supplier market. Many practices with similar offers compete for a limited number of patients.

It may happen that some patients leave and choose another practice. If the number of leavers becomes bigger than the number of new patients the dentist has to wonder about some modifications of the concept.

In the majority of cases any shortcomings relate to "soft" service, which are difficult to see from the perspective of the provider. Usually a lost patient doesn't leave any message explaining reasons for choosing a competitor. Riley et al. found that "there was a substantial subset of cases in which dentists were not aware of dissatisfaction" (2014). Thus, ways must be found to get information about the grade of satisfaction from current patients.

Investments

The physical environment represents one part of service quality. It should give confidence in dental treatments. A "clean and hygienic appearance" and "up-to-date equipment" are must-be attributes (Chang and Chang, 2012).

To get information about the patient's perception of the equipment may be a main driver in decision making for or against new investments.

The examples mentioned above all need to measure service quality, but as there are different goals there are completely different approaches necessary to get adequate and useful results.

View from the Perspective of the Service Recipient

The Patient

Normally a patient is not able to evaluate the performance of a dental treatment. "All they're able to perceive is what they see and feel" (Trettenero, 2016).

That is the reason why **every patient has an own picture of service quality**.

Different factors of the service bundle are of varying value for each one. To express this, Lewis and Booms (1983) noted that "service quality is a measure of how well the service level delivered matches customer expectations".

There are several ways to build these expectations:

9

- Innate feeling for quality, scientifically depicted as transcendent approach to quality (Shirley, 2011)
- Physical needs like tooth-ache
- Previous experiences
- Recommendations from family members and friends
- Social media, like rating platforms

The number of possible sources indicates the complexity of expectations, but one point is essential: A correct state-of-the-art treatment (following dental quality guidelines as mentioned above) is always assumed, there are other factors to differentiate service quality. In addition, these factors vary depending on dental subdivisions, which makes an evaluation difficult for a general dentist. A short poll (Appendix 1) conducted among 100 patients of a general dental practice shows the following result:

	Most important		Not sure		Least important
Examinations, Prophylaxis	Punctuality	Cost	Empathy	Duration	Low-Pain Treatment
Restorative Dentistry	Low-Pain Treatment	Aesthetics	Punctuality	Empathy	Duration
Prosthodontics, Implantology	Aesthetics	Cost	Low-Pain Treatment	Empathy	Punctuality
Oral Surgery	Empathy	Low-pain Treatment	Punctuality	Duration	Aesthetics
Pain Consultation	Low-Pain Treatment	Empathy	Duration	Aesthetics	Punctuality

Table 3

These are just a few random examples of service quality factors, but their distribution explains the challenge. (A more detailed list of general "Determinants of Service Quality" is published by Parasuraman et al. (1985).)

The challenge for a dentist lies in a **prediction of the patient's evaluation of the service in advance**. That would enable a good choice of factors to improve or to "influence these evaluations" (Gronroos, 1982).

This is aggravated by the fact that patients often really don't know what is individually possible and what to expect.

As the service "dentistry" is inseparable, the patient becomes part of it and influences the quality of the outcome. Normally she/he isn't aware of the impact of additional medical problems like allergies or medications, in- or decreased salivation or restricted mouth opening. That leads to unrealistic expectations and may be reflected in ridiculous evaluations.

Part 3: Methods to Measure Service Quality

The previous chapter identified the challenges of measuring service quality, now some suitable methods will be discussed.

The first step has to be a decision about the goal to get a clear view of **"what to measure"**. Then a suitable method for **"how to measure"** should be chosen.

Measuring Performance

Targets

These may be set for objectives and then be compared with existing data calculated by the practice IT. For some factors like numbers or size of fillings and their failures such a process is demanded by a mandatory quality management for dental practices (ZÄK-NR, 2018). Primarily it is a method to determine quantities, a special hypothesis (setting minimum failures or maximum numbers of performance) would be able to translate outcomes into statements about quality.

Measuring Perception

Surveys

It is possible to finish each treatment with a more or less detailed questionnaire about the patient's satisfaction. Results give an overview about the quantity of satisfied patients each week/month.

There are at least 3 problems to mention:
- This, too, states information about quantity.
- As every patient rates quality in different ways no generally accepted statement may be extracted.
  To get in depth information it would be necessary to interview each patient to learn how she/he expects service quality. (not feasible for a practice)
- The information is given after the treatment. Some patients may be lost as their perception cannot be influenced in advance (Gronroos, 1982).

SERVQUAL Model

This is the most widely accepted model developed by Parasuraman et al. (1985, 1988) "for assessing customer perceptions of service quality", which differs from objective quality and is viewed as "discrepancy between consumers' perception and expectations" (Parasuraman et al., 1988). It consists of a 22-item questionnaire to measure 5 dimensions used by customers to form expectations about and perceptions of service (Parasuraman et al., 1988):

- Reliability
- Assurance
- Tangibles
- Empathy
- Responsiveness

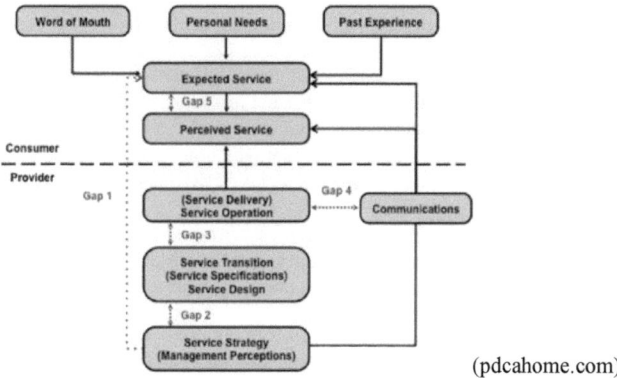

(pdcahome.com)

As the diagram shows, the model reveals 5 gaps, which may affect customers' perception:

Gap 1	Customer expectations vs. Company perceptions of customer expectations
Gap 2	Company perceptions of customer expectations vs. customer-driven service specifications (research)
Gap 3	Customer-driven service specifications vs. service delivery
Gap 4	Service delivery vs. Communications (external)
Gap 5	Perceived service vs. expected service f(Gap1, Gap2, Gap3, Gap4) (Parasuraman et al., 1985)

Table 4

SERVQUAL was developed using 4 service categories for investigation: retail banking, credit card, securities brokerage, and product repair and maintenance (Parasuraman et al., 1985). Does it really work with a complex service like "dentistry", too?

Before applying the instrument to dentistry two groups of criticism have to be discussed (Buttle, 1996):

1. Theoretical Parts
- The paradigmatic basis on the disconfirmation model (Oliver, 1980) is most questioned issue (Kulasin and Fortuny-Santos, 2005).
- The model doesn't "draw on previous social science research" (Andersson, 1992).
- Satisfaction as short-term experience is measured instead of long-term service quality (Cronin and Taylor, 1992).
 - This is important for a use in dentistry. If the questionnaire is completed immediately after treatment the patient will rate rather satisfaction than quality. To get clearer information follow-up surveys would be necessary. (not feasible for a practice)
- Evidence for relevance of the expectations-performance gap as basis for measuring service quality is missing (Cronin and Taylor, 1992). Difference scores are notoriously unreliable (Iacobucci et al., 1994).
 - A dental practice isn't interested in absolute numbers, the tendency counts.
- Focus lies on the process of service delivery, not the outcomes of the service encounter.
 - As outlined at "perishability" and the "product-based view on quality" the outcome is an important part of dental service quality. Even a perfect fulfilment of the 5 dimensions doesn't guarantee a perfect outcome. That is a category which should be added for dental use. Furthermore, an augmented model with both process and outcome components is a better predictor of consumer choice (Richard and Allaway, 1993).
- Predetermination of 5 dimensions doesn't work over all service sectors.
   Researchers found varying numbers depending on the service being offered (Babakus and Boller, 1992). It starts with 1 factor (utility company) (Babakus et al., 1993) and increases to 9 (hospital) (Carman, 1990).
 - In addition to "outcome" the dimension "patient" plays an important role. As mentioned above the patient's (medical) preconditions may influence outcome and perception of the process. As it is the patient, who completes the questionnaire, it may be difficult to create appropriate questions. Asking for premedication, general health and mood could offer a coefficient to critically weigh the results of the other dimensions.

2. Operational Parts
- Expectations are just a vague basis (Teas, 1993a); sometimes difficult to record (Carman, 1990). There may be several interpretations used by respondents, like importance, forecasted or deserved performance (Teas, 1993b).
 - An adapted choice of questions may narrow down problems in this field.
- The 7-point Likert scale may cause patients to use only extreme ends, because 2 to 6 aren't labelled (Lewis, 1993).
 - This point should be solved individually by labelling at least the midpoint.
- The completion of 2 questionnaires (pre-service and past-encounter) may be boring and confusing (Bouman and van der Wiele, 1992).
 - Especially dental patients aren't interested in completing 2 questionnaires. A suitable way could be a single one with scales for expectation and perception (Lewis, 1993) or a direct measure of the gap with one answer (perception was ... better-equal-worse... than expectation) (Carman, 1990).
   To avoid a second questionnaire and expectations the critics Cronin and Taylor (1992) introduced SERVPERF, based only on the SERVQUAL perception items.

The examples of criticism present a picture of imperfection of SERVQUAL. But most of them play no role in dentistry. Parasuraman et al. tried to create a model usable for all kinds of services. Applied as a framework with specific modifications it is very valuable in dentistry.

1. Working with the gap-model opens the eyes for potential improvements.

Gap 1	A dentist may believe modern equipment alone leads to a positive perception
Gap 2	Though there is high demand for professional tooth cleaning no staff is available to perform or no additional rooms can be provided
Gap 3	It is a challenge for assistants and dentists to work at a constantly high service level
Gap 4	Sometimes the dental team and patients speak different "languages"
Gap 5	The quintessence: Perception may be influenced, if expectations are known

Table 5

Especially communication is crucial.
- Usually there is no one right treatment to solve a dental case, there are several possibilities differing in time, price, or aesthetic. A patient appreciates an unbiased advice. Sometimes she/he is unable to communicate the problem, which makes a satisfying solution difficult.
- Realistic information about waiting time, treatment duration, pain, or costs will contribute to a positive perception.

2. Depending on the goal of the assessment the number of dimensions and items may be modified.

Current research in dental service quality shows examples with just 2 dimensions, but 90 questions (Dewi et al., 2011) or 30 (Bahadori et al., 2015) to 32 items (Adebayo et al., 2014), but the standard questionnaire is used, too (Mohebifar et al., 2016).

Interestingly, before the presentation of SERVQUAL a measurement tool only for dentistry was published (Davies and Ware, 1981).
The DSQ (Dental Satisfaction Questionnaire) identified 5 scales (dimensions) using 19 items:

Access	Time to get an appointment, waiting time at the office, office hours
Availability Convenience	Location, how to reach an office, parking lots, public transport conditions, Handicapped accessible
Cost	Fees, avoiding unnecessary expenses
Pain	Concern about pain
Quality	Treatment with respect checking everything

Table 6

A 5-point labelled scale is used to sum up a score.
As there are many parallels to SERVQUAL, this tool is criticised and refined over the years, too. So, there were 4 items added to cover the influence of team members (Chu and Lo, 1999). A focus on infection control and perceived skills of the dentists is added by Luo et al. (2018).

Conclusion

As the dental healthcare market is patient-driven today, a practice needs to stand out of the crowd to ensure economic success. Especially services of general practitioners are comparable. So, it would be a good choice to convince patients with high service quality. Unfortunately, this term cannot be generally defined, what makes it difficult to measure it. This report has outlined the challenges a practice owner may face. It is apparent from their array how to produce good results anyway.

1. Decision what to measure:
   Performance or outcomes, not affected by a patient's expectation
   or
   Perception of the treatment, affected by expectation

Since economic success depends on patients' satisfaction measuring quality from a patient's perspective makes most sense.

2. Difficulty to match a dentist's perspective – guided by definitions of professional bodies – with a patient's view
3. Prediction of the patient's evaluation of the service and therefore
4. How to measure something what is unknown as every patient has an own picture of quality

A widely accepted method to deal with these challenges is the SERVQUAL model. It defines service quality as a difference between perception and expectation.

As the patient completes the (second) questionnaire after a treatment, results cannot be influenced for that one, but a foundation for the future is established.

The SERVQUAL tool should be seen as a framework, that offers 5 dimensions and 22 items. Depending on own goals of research the number of them may be changed to set focal points. In that way the instrument is useful to assess parts of the treatment range or the overall performance of the practice.

Though SERVQUAL is criticised frequently in literature most of the arguments aren't important for practical use in dentistry.

Nevertheless, SERVQUAL is not the only solution to measure service quality.

To start with DSQ may be an easier way, as it was specifically developed for dentistry. Many practice owners are more familiar with the dimensions and items used there.

For marketing experts among dentists a combination of the two models create valuable results.

To conduct a questionnaire about quality seems to be relatively complex, but outcomes are really helpful. They give information about strengths and weaknesses of all parts of a practice and offer advice where to improve to get or keep a competitive advantage over other practices.

References

Adebayo, E.T., Adesina, B.A., Ahaji, L.E., Hussein, N.A. (2014) Patient assessment of the quality of dental care services in a Nigerian hospital, Journal of Hospital Administration 3(6), pp 20 – 28

Andersson, T.D. (1992) Another model of service quality: a model of causes and effects of service quality tested on a case within the restaurant industry, Quality Management in Service (Eds. Kunst, P. and Lemmink, J.) van Gorcum, The Netherlands, pp 41 – 58

Babakus, E. and Boller, G.W. (1992) An empirical assessment of the SERVQUAL scale, Journal of Business Research 24, pp 253 – 258

Babakus, E., Pedrick, D.L., Inhofe, M. (1991) Empirical examination of a direct measure of perceived service quality using SERVQUAL items, unpublished manuscript, Memphis State University, TN

Bahadori, M., Raadabadi, M., Ravangard, R., Baqldacchino, D. (2015) Factors affecting dental service quality, International Journal of Health Care Quality Assurance 28(7), pp 678 - 689

Baldwin, A. and Sohal, A. (2003) Service quality factors and outcomes in dental care, Managing Service Quality 13(3), pp 207 – 216

Bateson, J.E.G. (1995) Managing Service Marketing, Text and Readings, The Dryden Press, Fort Worth, TX

Bouman, M. and van der Wiele, T. (1992) Measuring service quality in the car service industry: building and testing an instrument, International Journal of Service Industry Management 3(4), pp 4 - 16

BusinessDictionary "Service", accessed at http://www.businessdictionary.com/definition/service.html on Oct. 13th 2018

Buttle, F. (1996) SERVQUAL: review, critique, research agenda, European Journal of Marketing 30(1), pp 8 – 32

Cambridge Dictionary (1983)"Performance" accessed at https://dictionary.cambridge.org/dictionary/english/performance on Oct. 13th2018

Carman, J.M. (1990) Consumer perceptions of service quality: an assessment of the SERVQUAL dimensions, Journal of Retailing 66 (1), pp 33 - 35

Chang, W.-J. and Chang, Y.-H. (2012) Patient satisfaction analysis: Identifying key drivers and enhancing service quality of dental care, Journal of Dental Sciences 10.006, pp 239 – 247

Chu, CH. And Lo, EC. (1999) Patients' satisfaction with dental servicesprovided by a university in Hong Kong, International Dental Journal 49(1), pp 53 - 59
Cronin, JJ.Jr and Taylor, S.A. (1992) Measuring service quality: a re-examination and extension, Journal of Marketing 56(7), pp 55 - 68

Crosby, P.B. (1979) Quality is free, McGraw-Hill, New York, NY

Davies, A.R. and Ware, J.E. (1981) Measuring Patient Satisfaction with Dental Care, Social Science and Medicine 15(6), pp 751 - 760

Dewi, F.D., Sudjana, G., Oesman, Y.M. (2011) Patient satisfaction analysis on service quality of dental health care based on empathy and responsiveness, Dental Research Journal 8(4), pp 172 – 177

DQA (2016), Quality Measurement in Dentistry, accessed at http://www.ada.org/~/media/ADA/Science%20and%20Research/Files/DQA_2016_Quality_Measurement_in_Dentistry_Guidebook.pdf?la=en on Oct 7[th2018]

Garvin, D.A. (1983) Quality on the line, Harvard Business Review 61, pp 64 - 75

Gronroos, C. (1982) Strategic Management and Marketing in the Service Sector, Marketing Science Institute, Cambridge, MA

Gronroos, C. (1990) Service Management: A Management Focus for Service Competition, International Journal of Service Industry Management 1(1), pp 6 - 14

Gronroos, C. (2007) Service Management and Marketing: Customer management in service competition, John Wiley, Chichester

Iacobucci, D., Grayson, K.A., Omstrom, A.L. (1994) The calculus of service quality and customer satisfaction: theoretical and empirical differentiation and integration, Advances in Service Marketing and Management (Eds. Swartz, T.A., Bowen, D.E., Brown, S.W.) 3 JAI Press, Greenwich, CT, pp 1 - 68

Kotler, P. and Armstrong, G. (1996) Principles of Marketing, Pearson, D.A. Prentice Hall International editions

KZBV Jahrbuch 2017, accessed at https://www.kzbv.de/jahrbuch-2017.768.de.html on Oct. 14th 2018

Kulasin, D. and Fortuny-Santos, J. (2005) Review oft he SERVQUAL Concept, 4[th]Research/expert Conference with International Participation „Quality 2005", Fojnica

Lewis, B.R. (1993) Service quality measurement, Marketing Intelligence and Planning 11 (4), pp 4 - 12

Lewis, R.C. and Booms, B.H. (1983) The Marketing Aspects of Service Quality, Emerging Perspectives on Services Marketing (Eds. Berry, L., Shostak, G., Upah, G.), Chicago, pp 99 – 107

Luo, J.Y.N., Liu, P.P., Wong, M.C.M. (2018) Patients' satisfaction with dental care: a qualitative study to develop a satisfaction instrument, BMC Oral Health 18:15

Mohebifar, R., Hasani, H., Barikani, A., Rafiei, S. (2016) Evaluating Service Quality from Patients' Perceptions: Application of Importance-performance Analysis Method, Osong Public Health Res Prospect 7(4), pp 233 – 238

Oliver, R.L. (1980) A cognitive model of the antecedents and consequences of satisfaction decisions, Journal of Marketing Research 17(11), pp 460 - 469

Parasuraman, A., Zeithaml, V., Berry, L.L. (1985) A Conceptual Model of Service Quality and Its Implications for Future Research, Journal of Marketing 49(4), pp 41 – 50

Parasuraman, A., Zeithaml, V., Berry, L.L. (1988) SERVQUAL: A Multiple-Item Scale for Measuring Consumer Perceptions of Service Quality, Journal of Retailing 64(1), pp 12 – 40

Pirsig, R. (1976) Zen and the Art of Motorcycle Maintenance, William Morrow and Company (Harper Collins), USA

Richard, M.D. and Allaway, A.W. (1993) Service quality attributes and choice behavior, Journal of Service Marketing 7(1), pp 59 - 68

Riley, J.L., Gordan, V.V., Hudak-Boss, S.E., Fellows, J.L., Rindal, D.B., Gilbert, G.H. (2014) Concordance between patient satisfaction and the dentist's view, JADA 145(4), pp 355 -362

Shirley, D. (2011) Project Management for Healthcare, CRC Press Taylor & Francis Group, Boca Raton, Fl

Teas, K.R. (1993a) Expectations, performance evaluation and consumers' perception of quality, Journal of Marketing 57(4), pp 18 – 24

Teas, K.R. (1993b) Consumer expectations and the measurement of perceived quality, Journal of Professional Service Marketing 8(2), pp 33 - 53

Trettenero, D.S. (2016) Quality dentistry: What does that really mean?, DentistryIQ, accessed at dentistryiq.com on Oct. 20th 2018

ZÄK-NR (2018) Quality Management accessed at portal.zaek-nr.de (protected area)

Zeithaml, V. (1981) How Consumer Evaluation Processes differ between Goods and Services, Marketing of Services (Eds. Donnelly, J. and George, W.), Chicago, pp 186 - 190

Tables

1a - d	Quality Approaches (user-, value-, manufacturing-, product-based)
2	STEEEP Quality
3	Poll about importance of service quality factors
4	SERVQUAL Gap 1 - 5
5	Dental Interpretation of SERVQUAL Gap 1 - 5
6	DSQ Dimensions

Pictures

Accessed from
- stepsnstages.com, Ortiz, J., 2018
- youtube.com, Sood, M., 2013
- acieta.com
- mbaknol.com
- ada.org
- ausenergy.com
- pdcahome.com

Appendix 1

Poll about service quality (at own dental practice)

Please rate the following factors in ascending order
(1 = least important – 5 = most important, 0 = no importance) for each subdivision:

	Aesthetic outcome	Cost	Duration of treatment	Empathy	Low-pain treatment	Punctuality
Examinations Prophylaxis						
Restorative Dentistry						
Prosthodontics Implantology						
Oral Surgery						
Pain Consultations						

Aesthetic outcome
Cost
Duration of treatment
Empathy
Low-pain treatment
Punctuality

YOUR KNOWLEDGE HAS VALUE

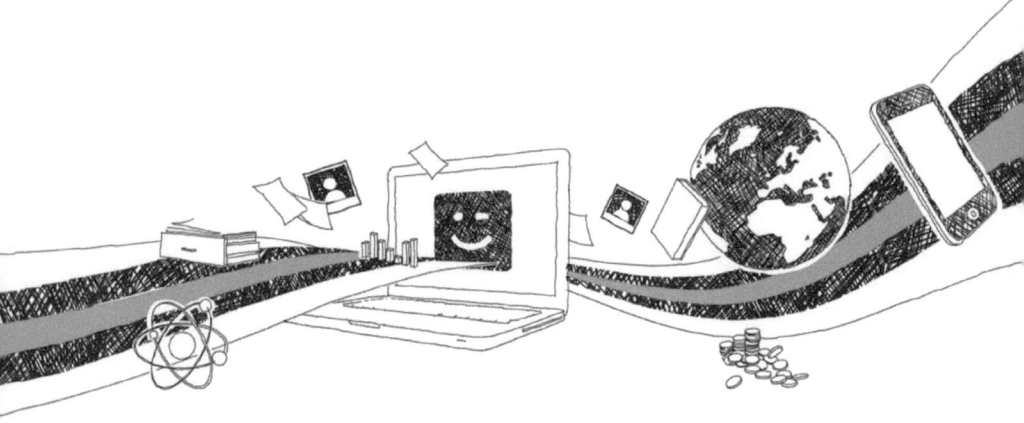

- We will publish your bachelor's and master's thesis, essays and papers

- Your own eBook and book - sold worldwide in all relevant shops

- Earn money with each sale

Upload your text at www.GRIN.com
and publish for free

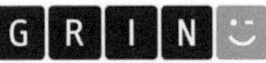